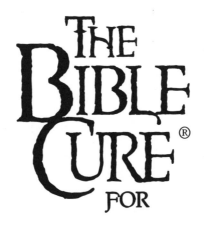

THE BIBLE CURE® FOR

ADD AND HYPERACTIVITY

DON COLBERT, M.D.

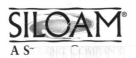

SILOAM®

A S

10661218

THE BIBLE CURE FOR ADD AND HYPERACTIVITY
by Don Colbert, M.D.
Published by Siloam
A Strang Company
600 Rinehart Road
Lake Mary, Florida 32746
www.strangdirect.com

Unless otherwise noted, all Scripture quotations are from the Holy Bible, New Living Translation, copyright © 1996. Used by permission of Tyndale House Publishers, Inc., Wheaton, Illinois 60189.

Scripture quotations marked NAS are from the New American Standard Bible. Copyright © 1960, 1962, 1963, 1968, 1971, 1972, 1973, 1975, 1977 by the Lockman Foundation. Used by permission. (www.Lockman.org)

Scripture quotations marked NCV are from The Holy Bible, New Century Version. Copyright © 1987, 1988, 1991 by Word Publishing, Dallas, Texas 75039. Used by permission.

Scripture quotations marked NKJV are from the New King James Version of the Bible. Copyright © 1979, 1980, 1982 by Thomas Nelson, Inc., publishers. Used by permission.

Copyright © 2001 by Don Colbert, M.D.
All rights reserved

Library of Congress Catalog Card Number: 00-112296
International Standard Book Number:
978-0-88419-744-7

This book is not intended to provide medical advice or to take the place of medical advice and treatment from your personal physician. Readers are advised to consult their own doctors or other qualified health professionals regarding the treatment of their medical problems. Neither the publisher nor the author takes any responsibility for any possible consequences from any treatment, action or application of medicine, supplement, herb or preparation to any person reading or following the information in this book. If readers are taking prescription medications, they should consult with their physicians and not take themselves off of medicines to start supplementation without the proper supervision of a physician.

08 09 10 11 12 — 16 15 14 13 12
Printed in the United States of America

ADD Is
Treatable and Beatable

God has promised greatness for your children. The Bible says, "How blessed is the man who fears the LORD, who greatly delights in His commandments. His descendants will be mighty on earth" (Ps. 112:1–2, NAS).

If your child shows signs of attention-deficit disorder (ADD), you may struggle to believe this statement, even though it's in the Bible. ADD behaviors can fray the nerves and test the hopes of the hardiest of parents.

If your child has ADD, you do not have to resort to heavy drug treatments that affect the unique, God-given personality of your precious child. Through practical natural methods, faith, prayer and God's Word, your ADD child can live a perfectly normal life free from the harmful effects of long-term drug treatments.

"Does My Child Have ADD?"

Do you suspect that your child may have ADD? Has a teacher or friend suggested it, but you just don't know for sure? Only your doctor can make a final diagnosis. Nevertheless, here are some questions to help you to understand if your child is struggling with attention-deficit disorder.

- Does he make too many careless mistakes with schoolwork and other activities?

- Does he have difficulty paying attention to tasks and play activities?

- Does he seem to not be listening, even when you speak directly to him?

- Does he fail to follow through on instructions and to finish homework, chores or other tasks?

If you see your youngster, or even an older child or adult, with these behaviors, your loved one may be silently struggling with the painful effects of ADD. I will offer a more detailed test later in this booklet.

About 3 to 5 percent of school-aged children have ADD or ADHD. ADD is attention-deficit disorder, and ADHD stands for attention-deficit hyperactivity disorder. Three times more boys experience hyperactivity than girls, while about the same number of boys and girls experience ADD without hyperactivity.

A Bold, New Approach

Even if you are almost certain that your loved one has ADD, don't fear. Your youngster does not have to suffer with the low self-esteem and poor grades common to many ADD sufferers.

With the help of the practical and faith-inspiring wisdom contained in this Bible Cure booklet, your loved one with ADD will fulfill his promise in God and be mighty in the earth. Through a natural approach that includes good nutrition, healthy lifestyle choices, vitamins and supplements, and most importantly of all, through the power of dynamic faith, you can halt the frustrating and debilitating symptoms of ADD.

Poor grades and low self-esteem are not your youngster's destiny. With God's grace, your child will be a powerful winner, achieving his potential in God with competence, success and joy!

As you read this book, prepare to overcome

the fear, painful low self-esteem and failure of ADD. This Bible Cure booklet is filled with practical steps, hope, encouragement and valuable information on how to develop a healthy, empowered lifestyle. In this book you will

*uncover God's divine plan of health
for body, soul and spirit
through modern medicine, good nutrition
and the medicinal power
of Scripture and prayer.*

As you read, apply and trust God's promises, you will also uncover powerful Bible Cure prayers to help you line up your thoughts and feelings with God's plan of divine health for you—a plan that includes living victoriously. In this Bible Cure booklet, you will find powerful insight in the following chapters:

You can confidently take the natural and

spiritual steps outlined in this book to control and overcome ADD forever.

It is my prayer that these practical suggestions for health, nutrition and fitness will bring wholeness to your life—body, soul and spirit. May they deepen your fellowship with God and strengthen your ability to worship and serve Him.

—DON COLBERT, M.D.

A Bible Cure Prayer
FOR YOU

Mighty God, You have promised that You will help my children to be mighty, successful people on this earth. I commit them to You—their lives, their futures, their successes and failures, their emotions and needs. I ask You to make them mighty in all they do. Give them the power to overcome every symptom of attention-deficit disorder and to live lives free from its debilitating effects. Amen.

Chapter 1

Understanding ADD

When you look to God for help, He promises to deliver your children from everything that would harm them—including attention-deficit disorder! The Bible says, "You can be very sure that the evil man will not go unpunished forever. And you can also be very sure that God will rescue the children of the godly" (Prov. 11:21, TLB).

To overcome ADD, it's important to first gain wisdom about it. The Scriptures say, "Wisdom is a tree of life to those who embrace her; happy are those who hold her tightly" (Prov. 3:18). This Bible cure response to ADD is founded upon a wise understanding of this disease, its root causes and its symptoms. Let's take an in-depth look at attention-deficit disorder and gain wisdom about it.

ADD behavior causes children to stand out among their classmates. They jump up and down from their seats, interrupt the teacher, talk out of turn and may treat other children and even teachers in inappropriate ways, hitting, cutting into lines and yanking away toys and school supplies.

Generally ADD is diagnosed when a child begins first or second grade. If it is not treated early in a child's life, 50 percent of ADD kids will usually struggle to be successful in school. They will fail grades and may eventually drop out of school without ever discovering the extent of their own intelligence or realizing the promise of their lives.

Many parents expect the symptoms of ADD to simply disappear as their children grow older. But children with ADD seldom outgrow their symptoms. Most ADD children grow up to become ADD teens, losing only the hyper-activity component through the maturing process. ADD teens continue to carry the traits of this disease into adulthood.

> *When I was a child, I spoke and thought and reasoned as a child does. But when I grew up, I put away childish things.*
> —1 Corinthians 13:11

About one-fifth to one-fourth of ADD adolescents will wind up in trouble with the law because of ADD symptoms. ADD teens will get more speeding tickets and end up having four times as many accidents. That is why it's critically important to properly diagnose ADD as early as possible. The sooner ADD children are treated with diet, nutrition, behavior modification and learning skills, the better their chance of experiencing early success.

Trouble Paying Attention

The main characteristic of ADD is inattention. These children are not always inattentive, but they are usually just not appropriately attentive. In other words, they demonstrate a selective form of attention. They usually focus on the wrong things at the wrong time. If the child is interested in a subject or activity, he can focus. But if the material is boring, he finds it extremely difficult to stay on task. Many youngsters with ADD can focus intently on subjects or material they enjoy.

Children with ADD often sit in class and daydream, and thus many times they will miss out on important information. Such youngsters can create major problems for teachers who are trying to keep the children focused in a classroom. Inattentive ADD kids ask inappropriate questions when they tune back in, often disrupting the entire class.

This inattention carries over into the teenage years. Many ADD teens cannot keep a job because of their inability to concentrate and focus on complex tasks. Many people usually see the inattention as absentmindedness since ADD teens tend to tune in and tune out.

"I Want It Now!"—
ADD and Impulsiveness

ADD kids are notorious for wanting what they want when they want it. This kind of impulsivity is an earmark of ADD and ADHD children. These children act before they think. Unfortunately, ADD children, teenagers and even adults seldom consider consequences before they act. You can imagine the trouble this gets them into with parents, teachers and even the law.

"My Dog Ate It!"

"My dog ate my homework because he was so hungry after fighting the bobcats who were attacking me and keeping me from finishing!" Such tall tales are not uncommon to ADD children.

ADD youngsters and teens, driven by impulsivity and low self-esteem, are easily tempted to lie to parents, teachers and even bosses regarding their inappropriate behaviors. ADD children are known for fabricating outlandish stories in order to maintain their self-esteem. These children will impulsively tell lies to avoid punishment.

"Wanna Come Out and Play?"

Another characteristic of ADD is being easily distracted. Children with ADD are easily drawn away by anything they may see or hear. Many times children with ADD will start a task but lose interest and begin to do something else. At this point they may completely forget what the original task was. ADD children require constant supervision and encouragement to avoid getting sidetracked.

"That Child Is Hyper!"

Children are naturally full of energy, excitement and playfulness. So how do parents know when to consider a child who is a ball of energy abnormal?

Hyperactivity is another very common characteristic of ADD. Many children demonstrate hyperactivity in which they are more restless and active at inappropriate times. When other children are seated and listening, these children are restless and fidgety, tapping a pencil on their desk like a drum, dancing around, playing with anything nearby or clowning around to attract attention. A child with hyperactivity and ADD is much more disruptive at school and at home than a child with just ADD.

Angry teachers, failed tests, poor grades and disappointed parents can crush a small ADD or ADHD child. Since it is difficult to develop a good self-image when you're failing at school, these youngsters quickly develop very low self-esteem.

> *In that day the wolf and the lamb will live together; the leopard and the goat will be at peace. Calves and yearlings will be safe among lions, and a little child will lead them all.*
> —Isaiah 11:6

It's not easy for children with ADD to make and keep friends since other children usually view them as annoying. Often the brunt of jokes and usually left out of games, they begin life with painful rejection and deep isolation, which crushes them even more.

Therefore, it is critically important to intervene

in the lives of ADD and ADHD youngsters before the internal and external pressure surrounding this disorder causes a pattern of failure and low self-esteem.

ADD and ADHD

ADD can occur with or without hyperactivity. ADD with hyperactivity is also called ADHD, or attention-deficit hyperactivity disorder.

Children with ADD who are not hyperactive can often go undiagnosed. These youngsters may be diagnosed when they are much older and begin failing in school. Parents and teachers can label these youngsters as lazy and lacking in ambition and motivation.

ADD Boredom

School feels painfully boring to ADD students. Reading seems so tedious that it may put them to sleep. They also fall asleep during class lectures or when doing homework. ADD kids need stimulating activities such as computer games, videos and TVs to hold their attention and interest.

Most ADD kids live in a foggy state of drowsiness or underarousal nearly all of the time. They are extremely forgetful and unreliable. They are very poor listeners and have an extremely hard time following verbal instructions in class or at home.

The Bible Cure prescription at the end of this chapter contains questions that will help you to assess whether or not your youngster or young adult has ADD or ADHD.

Most importantly, don't fear. Remember God's promise to rescue your children and to make them great. Some of the greatest men and women who have ever lived struggled with ADD or ADHD. Among them are Thomas Edison and Winston Churchill.

Your frustration and disappointment may feel overwhelming at times, but I promise you that if you look to God, He will not fail you. He created your son or daughter with a marvelous destiny.

> *He said to them, "Let the children come to me. Don't stop them! For the Kingdom of God belongs to such as these."*
> —MARK 10:14

And He will help your child to achieve that calling. He is so faithful. Even though it may be difficult for you to imagine, He loves your child much more than you do! With God's help, your struggle with ADD or ADHD will only make you better, stronger, more compassionate and caring people.

There is no challenge that's bigger than God, and He has promised to see your family through this. "For God has said, 'I will never fail you. I will never forsake you'" (Heb. 13:5). If you look to Him, you will not be disappointed.

A Bible Cure Prayer
For You

Dear heavenly Father, You are my child's heavenly Father, and I know You love my child and are more committed to his success and happiness than I am. I give You all my fear, discouragement and frustration over ADD and ADHD. I ask You to help our family walk Your path to deliverance, peace, hope and healing. I thank You ahead of time, by faith, for bringing our family through this and for blessing our child with future success. Amen.

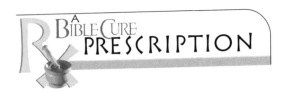

A BIBLE CURE PRESCRIPTION

Does Your Child Have ADD?

Fill out this ADD/ADHD quiz to find out if your child or loved one may have ADD or ADHD. (The symptoms must have started before age seven and must have been evident for six months.)

Check the appropriate boxes.

Inattention

❏ Often fails to give close attention to details or makes careless mistakes in schoolwork, work or other activities

❏ Often has difficulty sustaining attention in tasks or play activities

❏ Often does not seem to listen when spoken to directly

❏ Often does not follow through on instructions and fails to finish schoolwork, chores or duties in the workplace

❏ Often has difficulty organizing tasks and activities

Hyperactivity

❑ Often fidgets with hands or feet or squirms in seat

❑ Often leaves seat in classroom or in other situations in which remaining seated is expected

❑ Often runs about or climbs excessively in situations in which it is inappropriate (in adolescents or adults, may be limited to subjective feelings of restlessness)

❑ Often has difficulty playing or engaging in leisure activities quietly

❑ Is often on the go or acts as if driven by a motor

If you have checked more than half of the boxes in either category, your child or loved one may be experiencing ADD or ADHD and should be evaluated by a professional.

NOTE: *The Diagnostic and Statistical Manual of Mental Disorders* identifies three types of ADHD: (1) predominantly hyperactive-impulsive type; (2) predominantly inattentive type; (3) ADHD combined type.[1]

Chapter 2

Lifestyle Solutions

Your children are God's wonderfully unique and immeasurably valuable creation. God gave them to you as a rich and great blessing. The Bible says, "Children are a gift from the LORD; they are a reward from him" (Ps. 127:3). It's God's purpose and plan for your life that these years of raising your children be filled with joy, wonder and excitement.

You don't have to let the trauma of ADD or ADHD ruin the blessings of these wonderful years. Let's take a look at some natural lifestyle solutions that can make all the difference to your family's sense of peace and joy.

Your Bright, Creative ADD Child

ADD and ADHD children are much brighter than

they are able to demonstrate on tests and in the classroom.

These youngsters are specially gifted with boundless energy and enthusiasm that can be harnessed and used to help them become extremely successful. Flexible and spontaneous, ADD kids are often extremely creative. The great inventor Thomas Edison demonstrated classic symptoms of ADD.

Their gifts are endless. Children with ADD are very entertaining, with quick wits and super senses of humor. Many of them have a special tenacity that helps them to never give up. Winston Churchill, Great Britain's well-loved prime minister, had ADD and hyperactivity. He was known for his great tenacity during World War II.

> *I assure you, anyone who doesn't have their kind of faith will never get into the Kingdom of God.*
> —Mark 10:15

Individuals with ADD have a truly unique and unusual way at looking at the world. They usually are able to see the big picture rather than merely a small part. Individuals with ADD tend to be much more intuitive, which allows them to perceive the true motives and intentions of others.

ADD children have their own truly unique way of thinking, behaving and learning, and they possess incredible gifts and talents that can make them highly successful in life.

The Trouble With Ritalin

Most physicians prescribe Ritalin to control the symptoms of ADHD. Nearly 85 percent of children with ADHD take Ritalin or similar drugs.

Ritalin is an amphetamine-type drug that speeds up the metabolism of adults. However, this drug tends to have the opposite effect on children. According to *The Merrow Report*, a quarterly PBS documentary, "by the year 2000 we'll be diagnosing and medicating 15 percent of our children, eight million kids."[1]

Ritalin and Addiction

According to the U.S. Drug Enforcement Agency, Ritalin is considered a Class II drug and a controlled substance, a fact that is not widely known. Other drugs in this same category are cocaine, methamphetamine and methadone. In many of today's classrooms, it is not uncommon for 25 percent of the students to be on Ritalin.[2]

Destructive Side Effects

The most common side effects of Ritalin are loss of appetite and muscle tics. A tic is any involuntary, regularly repeated, spasmodic contraction of a muscle. It may be a facial grimace or an involuntary movement of the head, hands or arms.

Other common side effects of Ritalin are insomnia, short-term growth retardation, anxiety, stomachaches, headaches and Ritalin rebound. Rebound occurs when Ritalin wears off, and some children actually become even more hyperactive than they were before starting the medicine. Others may become depressed.

Ritalin can be very helpful over the short term. But since it merely treats symptoms and does not address the root problems of the disease, you are better off to limit its use.

> *Teach your children to choose the right path, and when they are older, they will remain upon it.*
> —Proverbs 22:6

Drug therapy improves ADD and ADHD symptoms in 75 percent of young people. However, I believe there are much safer methods that we will be discussing throughout this booklet.

Television and the Role of Environment

There are more individuals with ADD in North America than in any other place in the world. This fact causes many psychologists to believe that environment plays a significant role.

Do you realize that, according to the American Psychological Association, children who watch two to four hours of TV a day witness about 8,000 murders and 100,000 other acts of brutality by the time they leave elementary school? That's a lot of stimulation for a young mind to cope with.

Limit Television Violence

Limit television and video games to about one hour a day during the school week and two to three hours on weekends. Electronic violence programs your children for failure. Never allow your young children to play violent video games or watch violence on TV. Use the VCR to record nonviolent children's programs on Saturday, and play them in the evenings. Sit down with your child once in a while and play nonviolent video games with him.

> *They will live in prosperity, and their children will inherit the Promised Land.*
> —Psalm 25:13

Parents of children with ADD and ADHD also need to understand their child's learning style. This will help a lot in controlling his ADD symptoms.

ADD and Learning Styles

Three main memory and learning types are common. Let's look at them.

Visual learners. Most people, nearly 65 percent, are visual learners. These learners picture what they need to remember in their heads. Charts, illustrations, graphs and highlighters are helpful learning tools for visual learners.

Visual learners usually learn more quickly than other learners and are able to better recall the material they have learned.

Auditory learners. Twenty percent of learners learn best through auditory or hearing means. Lectures, teaching cassettes, music and rhymes are vital memory tools for auditory learners.

Auditory learners are usually better at organizing complex material in their minds.

Kinesthetic learners. About 15 percent of us have kinesthetic memory styles. This is a very "hands-on" learning style. Kinesthetic learners memorize by actually doing whatever it is they're learning.

Our schools are not really set up for these learners. Kinesthetic learners love to work with their hands, and they need to move in order to learn. They learn best by role-playing, hands-on activities, physical games, drama or any activity that involves movement while learning.

> *Then he took the children into his arms and placed his hands on their heads and blessed them.*
> —Mark 10:16

Most individuals with ADD and ADHD are kinesthetic learners. Years ago young men and women learned through the kinesthetic method of apprenticeship, which simply meant studying under someone skilled in their trade. Young men assisted a carpenter or a blacksmith, or they worked with their fathers on the farm. Young women worked alongside of their mothers, aunts and grandmothers. Society was developed and passed down the generations through this hands-on learning style.

But today, this once shared learning method has been replaced by other learning styles that suit the academic subjects taught in schools. Nevertheless, ADD kinesthetic learners need hands-on experiences to succeed. Listening to lectures or watching the teacher write on the blackboard or on transparencies tend to bore ADD kids. But let them dig their hands into clay or dress up like a president, and they begin to shine.

A BIBLE CURE HEALTH TIP

Here are few suggestions for helping to create a better classroom environment for your ADD child:

- Visit your child's classroom during class to observe your child.

- Moving your child closer to the teacher and away from distractions can help him focus.

- What kind of temperament does his teacher have? Is she rigid, irritable? Does she seem to take her frustrations out on the children?

- Schedule regular periodic meetings with the teacher to discuss your child's special learning needs.

- Many schools permit parents to eat lunch with their children. Join your child regularly for lunch.

Getting Organized

Children with ADD or ADHD have the intelligence, but lack of organization usually prevents them from accomplishing their goals. Your ADD child needs your help to get organized, and getting organized will do wonders for helping your ADD child to relax and succeed.

First, get your young-ster's room organized. ADD children need to both clean and organize their rooms on a daily basis. Make this part of their daily chores. Since these children are notoriously disorganized, it's vitally important that you step in and help.

> *The godly always give generous loans to others, and their children are a blessing.*
> —Psalm 37:26

Ask your child's teacher to help him organize his desk every week. Although your ADD child may not be naturally inclined to organization, he can learn by getting into the daily habit of being organized.

Developing Regular Routines

ADD children desperately need regular routines and consistent rules. A structured environment is absolutely essential to their success. They should get up about the same time each morning and go to bed at about the same time each evening. They should have meals on a regular schedule at about the same time each day, and they should eat with other family members. These children need structure in the home, structure in the classroom and even structure while playing.

Keep an Assignment Book

A homework assignment book will be very helpful. Make sure that your child brings it home daily. You may need to get the teacher to fill it in at first until it becomes a habit. Forgetting or not doing homework is one of the main reasons that many ADD children make poor grades.

Meet with your child's teacher regularly to be sure he is bringing home assignments and completing them.

Minimize Distractions

Turn off the TV or radio and unplug the phone when your child is trying to study. Keeping all distracting noises to a minimum will help your ADD youngster to focus.

Get Ready for Tomorrow

Get your child ready for the school day the night before. Spend a few minutes together placing completed assignments into his backpack, helping him think about whether or not he'll need any other items such as gym clothes or special requests from the teacher and then laying out clothing for the next day.

Healthy, Wealthy and Wise

Get your ADD youngster to bed early—it's critically important that he gets at least eight hours of sleep at night. Many require nine or even ten hours of sleep.

Clear Expectations

Establish clear and consistent rules and expectations for children with ADD. Put the family rules on a colorful poster in the kitchen or on the refrigerator. Instead of having a lot of small rules, have a few key rules.

Successful Reader

Your ADD child will become a successful reader. Although reading may feel extremely boring to many children with ADD, this can be easily overcome.

Buy your child beautiful books with wonderful pictures to help him develop an excitement about books. Give books as a reward, and never, *never* associate reading with punishment. Treat your child to weekly visits to the library, read to him often and let him pick out books that draw his interest.

Conclusion

Your ADD child was created by God with his own truly unique and gifted style of learning, seeing and expressing himself in the world around him. He's bright, brimming with creative ideas and youthful energy. As you use natural and super-natural methods to develop, mold and shape his truly unique destiny, you will discover a treasure chest of delights in the personality and heart of your wonderful ADD child. Begin thanking God right now for the wisdom and grace to unlock his powerful potential.

A BIBLE CURE PRAYER
FOR YOU

Dear God, thank You for blessing my life and the lives of my family with my precious ADD child. Give me the wisdom and grace to appreciate the truly unique and gifted person that You created my child to be. Help me to use all of these Bible cure steps to structure my child's life so all the potential within my ADD child is released in a life of joyful success. Amen.

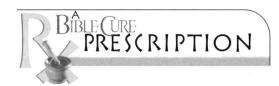

A BIBLE CURE
PRESCRIPTION

List the lifestyle changes that you intend to make.

_____

_____

_____

_____

_____

_____

Write a prayer thanking God for your child's future success.

_____

_____

_____

_____

_____

_____

_____

Chapter 3

Exercising Options

Begin building your ADD or ADHD child's future success by establishing fitness habits that will form a lasting foundation for his life. The Bible says, "Teach your children to choose the right path, and when they are older, they will remain upon it" (Prov. 22:6).

Physical activity plays an enormous role in the life of an ADD or ADHD youngster. Parents can use this to great advantage as a healthy and natural way of controlling ADD and ADHD. Let's take a look.

Sports and Exercise

Your child may seem to have a need to move about constantly, especially if he has ADHD. That may be great for football or basketball, but what about studying?

Well, who says your child always has to sit still

while studying? You may find that he actually studies better if allowed to pace back and forth or move in other ways.

Role-playing. Use role-playing games with him during study times. For instance, if you are studying spelling words, let him pretend to be contestant on *Jeopardy!* and give him a bell or a buzzer to ring when he has the right answer.

Field trips. If your child is studying animals, why not take him to a petting zoo where he can actually see and feel the subject?

If your daughter is studying math, let her make the change in a restaurant and hand it to the waitress.

Hands-on experiences. Remember your child is a hands-on learner. Whatever you can do to give feet to the experience of learning will make it real and practical. Something as simple as grabbing a Cheerios box and dumping it out to help with math questions can make all of the difference in the world.

Use a big map for geography and let your child find cities, countries and other sites and mark them with pins or stars. Felt boards and cut-out figures can also help to enrich your hands-on learner.

Pacing. ADD and ADHD kids often think better on their feet. Let your child walk or pace as he studies. After all, who ever said that all studying must be done sitting at a desk anyway?

You may find that your child can sit and concentrate easier if you mix hands-on "action learning" experiences with times of sitting quietly.

Posture. To help keep your child alert in the classroom and at home while studying, make sure that he maintains good posture.

Calming With Exercise

You may be convinced that sports and other activities do anything but calm down your ADHD or ADD child. Many parents resort to video games and television to try to quiet their busy youngsters.

Physical exercise is a much better approach. Let him participate in lots of sports, and provide regular, daily

> *This promise is to you and to your children.*
> —Acts 2:39

times of hard physical play. Basketball, baseball, football and soccer are great healthy channels for his boundless energy.

Your child's energy and strength are gifts to him from God. Let him come home from school and express as much of his energy through sports and physical activities as possible. You may feel that it only stirs up his engine, but eventually you will notice that he does begin to calm down and relax more. Over time you will begin to notice that he is calmer and more focused later on when it's time to do his studies.

Focusing Techniques

When your child begins school, you can start teaching him some valuable focusing techniques. Like exercising a muscle, attention span can be stretched and increased through training. Here are a few easy-to-learn focusing techniques that are sure to net powerful results.

External object technique. Have your child focus on an object such as a favorite toy, a picture, a cloud or some other object of interest. Get a stop watch, or watch the clock, and time how long he is able to focus on one object without talking, giggling or turning away.

Once your child has done this repeatedly and is able to do it for more than five to ten minutes, you can then teach your child to focus inwardly.

Internal focus technique. Have your child focus on a word such as *Jesus* or develop a belief such as "I am an excellent student." He can even focus on his own breathing. Have him take a deep breath, inhaling over about five seconds and then slowly exhaling over five seconds.

Work with your child on these techniques for about ten to twenty minutes every day. Before long you will notice that he begins to focus better while in class or while doing homework. Always have him focus on things of interest to him, and be sure to keep it fun. Be creative and make it a game.

You will notice that his mind will tend to wander off continually. Patiently and lovingly bring him back to the focus object. As distracting thoughts and daydreams compete for his mind, teach him to keep refocusing on the idea at hand. You are developing strong mental "muscles" that will carry his thoughts throughout college and career.

Biofeedback Techniques

One of the most exciting new treatments for ADD is brain wave biofeedback, otherwise known as neurofeedback. This form of biofeedback teaches how to concentrate and focus as an individual views a computer screen. By controlling a bar graph on the computer screen, your ADD youngster can then produce brain waves that help to maintain focus and attention. Through repeated practice the ADD sufferer eventually will become able to produce these attentive brain waves on their own.

Doctor Joel Lubar is one of the nation's foremost authorities on ADHD neurofeedback treatment. Of the patients whom he has treated, more than 90 percent have responded well to neurofeedback.[1]

> *The children*
> *of your people*
> *will live in security.*
> *Their children's*
> *children will thrive*
> *in your*
> *presence.*
> —Psalm 102:28

As a child begins to exercise the brain pathways that control attention, he experiences how it feels to finally concentrate. This means he can now differentiate between when he is concentrating and when he is drifting off.

Conclusion

Don't you wish you had the energy and creativity that your child has? It takes just a tank of gas to drive to the next state, but it takes a rocket full of fuel to go to the moon. Your child may have more energy than most kids, but he also has the fuel to go farther. Remember that rockets are really nothing more than extremely well-channeled explosions.

Commit today to help your child channel his energy, his enthusiasm and his zest for life, to help him reach beyond the stars. It may seem

> *Those who fear the Lord are secure; he will be a place of refuge for their children.*
> —Proverbs 14:26

like an impossible challenge at first, but with God's help, you and your ADD child will go all the way!

A BIBLE CURE PRAYER
FOR YOU

*Dear Lord, help me to always be thankful
for the one-of-a-kind individual my child
is and for the gift of boundless energy and
enthusiasm with which You blessed him.
Give me creative ways to structure his
activities and chores so that his physical
life will be perfectly suited to the wonderfully unique person You made him. Help
me to train him up in the way he should
go. Amen.*

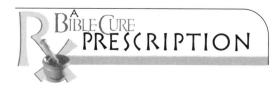

A BIBLE CURE PRESCRIPTION

What creative ways can you think of to make your child's homework time a more hands-on experience?

_____

_____

_____

Create a schedule of your child's daily routine that provides plenty of very structured time for exercise, activities and for creative expressions in homework.

_____

_____

_____

_____

_____

_____

_____

Chapter 4

A Natural Nutritional Approach

God's rich love for your child includes blessing your youngster's life with natural, truly wholesome and nourishing foods. God says, "But I would feed you the best of foods. I would satisfy you with wild honey from the rock" (Ps. 81:16).

The very best diet is an essential part of your Bible cure for ADD. Healthy, nutritious food is a major component to your natural solution to ADD and ADHD.

An ADD Diet

Although most ADD is not caused directly by diet, what your child eats can definitely contribute to learning and behavioral problems.

Some researchers believe that ADD is caused by an imbalance of important chemicals in the brain called neurotransmitters. Diet can dramatically improve the amount and function of these neuro-transmitters. That's why good nutrition can help to improve both the behavior and learning of ADD kids.

These neurotransmitters need to be replenished on a daily basis. Therefore, adequate nutrition on a daily basis is especially critical for these children.

The Care and Feeding of Your Child's Brain

Several key neurotransmitters are critically important for focusing, learning and memory. These most important neurotransmitters include acetylcholine, norepinephrine, serotonin and dopamine. What your child eats every day forms these essential brain chemicals. Let's take a brief look at these powerful chemicals.

Acetylcholine is an incredible neurotransmitter and is the main brain chemical for thought and memory. You can actually restore your brain's level of acetylcholine in just a few hours by eating

> *Even children are known by the way they act, whether their conduct is pure and right.*
> —PROVERBS 20:11

certain nutrients such as lecithin. Foods highest in choline include the following:

- Egg yolks
- Wheat germ
- Soy beans
- Peanuts
- Natural peanut butter
- Whole-wheat products

The Brain Power of Protein

Foods that are high in protein help to form the neurotransmitters dopamine and norepinephrine. They come from amino acids found in the following high-protein foods:

- Seafood
- Soy
- Poultry
- Dairy products

Getting a Good Breakfast

High-protein foods supply a rich amount of certain amino acids, which eventually are converted in your body to norepinephrine and dopamine— two main brain-boosting chemicals.

To be sure that your ADD child is getting enough of the chemical punch that proteins provide, have him eat his meats, eggs, dairy products and other proteins first. Wait thirty minutes to an hour before you let him eat carbohydrate-rich foods. By eating like this, your youngster will absorb the highest amount of the amino acid phenylalanine, which will then be converted to the brain boosters norepinephrine and dopamine.

Often a high-protein diet will help ADD children to focus better.

Breakfast should be the most important high-protein meal. Get your ADD child started each morning with yogurt, eggs, lean breakfast meats such as soy sausage, soy cheese or a protein smoothie.

> *The godly walk with integrity; blessed are their children after them.*
> —PROVERBS 20:7

Serotonin for a Peaceful Child

Another powerful neurotransmitter is serotonin. Serotonin gives a feeling of well-being and contentment, and it helps us to fall asleep. This powerful chemical is manufactured in the body by eating foods that contain the amino acid tryptophan. Without eating the right foods, your body is unable to make adequate amounts of serotonin.

The safest way to get tryptophan is from dietary sources. Here's a list of foods rich in this powerful brain-boosting chemical:

- Turkey
- Milk
- Dairy foods
- Sunflower seeds
- Meat
- Bananas
- Most sugary foods and starches

Foods high in tryptophan tend to sedate the brain, whereas foods high in tyrosine and phenylalanine stimulate the brain. Children need more of these brain-stimulating amino acids in the morning and at noon when they need to focus and learn. They need more tryptophan in the evening when they need to calm down and go to sleep.

Craving Carbs

Eating carbohydrates such as a lot of fruit, starchy vegetables and sugary foods increase serotonin levels. In fact, people who crave carbohydrates and sugars often have a craving for the neurotransmitter serotonin.

Children with ADD or ADHD who eat a lot of carbohydrates and sugars will demonstrate more inattention, distractibility, problems focusing, spaciness and hyperactivity. They will usually then consume more sugars and carbohydrates, further compounding the problem. Foods high in sugar and carbohydrates actually sedate the brain, which will decrease mental performance.

Sweet Thoughts—
Sugar and the Brain

The brain's exclusive source of fuel is glucose, or sugar. Without adequate glucose the brain doesn't function very well. Even though the brain is only about 2 percent of your total body weight, it uses about 20 percent of your energy.

Your brain's supply of glucose also has to be replenished frequently. If brain cells do not get enough glucose, an energy crisis occurs. The result is a disturbance in mood, behavior, concentration, attention span and memory. You can see that for a child's brain to function at optimal levels, it must get a constant supply of glucose from the blood. Either high or low levels will affect brain functioning.

When you are learning new skills or new information, or when you are solving a problem, your brain burns even more glucose. If your body's reserves are not replenished by eating the right kind of sugars and carbohydrates, memory, attention span, concentration and mood will all be affected.

To keep your blood sugar stabilized so that your brain can function at peak efficiency, you must eat certain carbohydrates that will cause a slow, gradual rise in blood sugar instead of highly processed carbohydrates that cause a rapid increase.

Carbohydrates that cause a rapid increase in blood sugar are known as carbohydrates with a high glycemic index. Carbohydrates with a slow gradual rise of blood sugar are known as carbohydrates with a low glycemic index.

High-glycemic foods. Foods with a high glycemic index stimulate the pancreas to secrete too much insulin. Believe it or not, this actually causes low blood sugar with symptoms including decreased attention span, hyperactivity, spaciness and learning difficulties.

Foods with a high glycemic index initially cause the blood sugar to shoot up. But then this rise in blood sugar signals the pancreas that the body has too much sugar. The pancreas then secretes insulin to bring the blood sugar level back down. This excessive release of insulin actually causes the blood sugar to become low.

Low-glycemic foods. However, low-glycemic foods do not cause excessive amounts of insulin to flood into your body. Therefore, your blood sugar remains more stable without the highs and lows.

Your ADD child will find it easier to focus and learn when provided with low-glycemic carbohydrates.

What kinds of food are considered high-glycemic foods? Processed starches such as white bread, rice cakes and white rice; even baked potatoes are very high. Eating these foods is the same as eating candy as far as your body is concerned. That's because they will trigger elevated insulin levels, which result in low blood sugar.

So you can see that simply avoiding sweets and sugars in your child's diet is not enough. Limit or avoid all high-glycemic foods. The more you are able to regulate your child's blood sugar and insulin, the better his brain will be able to work. Thus, your child will be better able to focus and learn.

Refuse Refined Sugars

The most important nutritional advice that I give all mothers of children with ADD and ADHD is to eliminate all refined sugars from the child's diet.

Here's a helpful list of high- and low-glycemic foods.

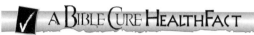

Glycemic Index of Foods

EXTREMELY HIGH (GREATER THAN 100)

Corn flakes
Millet
Potato, baked, instant
Honey

Rice, instant, puffed
Bread, French
Carrots, cooked

GLYCEMIC STANDARD=100 PERCENT

Bread, white

HIGH (80–100)

Bread, rye, wheat,
  whole meal
Grape Nuts
Muesli
Crispbread
Corn, sweet
Potato, broiled, mashed
Apricots
Banana
Mango
Pastry

Crackers
Shredded wheat
Tortilla, corn
Rice, brown, white
Raisins
Papaya
Candy bars
Cookies
Ice cream, low fat
Corn chips

MODERATELY HIGH (60–80)

Buckwheat
Bread, rye, pumpernickel
Macaroni, white
Yams
Green peas

All Bran
Bulgur
Spaghetti, white, brown
Sweet potatoes
Green peas (frozen)

Baked beans (canned) Kidney beans (canned)
Fruit cocktail   Grapefruit juice
Orange juice   Pineapple juice
Pears (canned)   Grapes
Oatmeal cookies   Potato chips
Sponge cake

Moderate (40–60)

White beans   Tomato soup
Green peas (dried)   Lima beans
Butter beans   Chickpeas (garbanzo)
Kidney beans   Black-eyed peas
Black beans   Apple juice
Orange   Apple
Pears   Milk
Yogurt

Low (less than 40)

Barley   Soybeans
Red lentils   Plums
Peaches   Peanuts
Fructose

Food Choices

Choosing foods to purchase and serve is a matter of habit—either a good one or a bad one. Getting into the habit of selecting and preparing foods with a moderate or low glycemic index will benefit your entire family, and it's not really that difficult. You can do it!

Whole fruit has a much lower glycemic index than juices. That means you should serve your ADD child a cut-up orange or apple instead of a glass of juice. That's simple enough.

Vegetables are great. They tend to have low glycemic indexes, and vegetables such as beans, legumes, peas and lentils are high in fiber and have lower glycemic indexes.

Whole grains and whole-grain cereals such as old-fashioned oatmeal, oat bran and high-fiber cereals have low glycemic indexes. Also, most dairy products have low glycemic indexes except for ice cream and fruit-filled yogurt. Plain yogurt with freshly sliced fruit is an excellent low-glycemic food.

Brain-Friendly Fats

Your ADD child needs the right kinds of fats for his brain and nervous system to function properly. About 30 percent of a child's calories must come from fat. Brain cells, as well as the protective covering around nerve cells, depend on a daily intake of essential fats and healthy fats in your child's diet.

Three Types of Bad Fat

To provide a natural, dietary solution for ADD, you need to understand the three types of fat:

- Saturated fats—the most harmful
- Polyunsaturated fats—the next most harmful
- Hydrogenated fats—the most dangerous

Saturated fats are found in all meats. But the highest concentrations are found in cheese, butter, lard, skins of chickens and fatty cuts of meat such as bacon and hamburgers.

Articles and television programs have been warning us for years that saturated fat contributes to heart disease by causing a buildup of plaque in the walls of the blood vessels. However, we seldom hear about the effect of saturated fats upon our brains. This dangerous fat also enters into every cell in the body, including brain cells.

When too much saturated fat enters a brain cell, it causes the cell walls to harden and thicken. This makes it difficult for cell walls to allow nutrients to come into the cell and to allow waste products to leave the cell. Once healthy brain cells can begin to struggle to function.

Polyunsaturated fats can damage brain cells,

too. These fats include safflower oil, sunflower oil, corn oil and soybean oil to name a few.

Polyunsaturated fats oxidize faster than saturated fats, creating free radicals. Take a bottle of polyunsaturated oil such as corn oil out of the refrigerator and leave it open on your kitchen counter. Very quickly this oil will become rancid. This oxidation also occurs in the body. When these polyunsaturated fats are oxidized, they create tremendous amounts of free radicals, which can damage and even destroy brain cells.

Hydrogenated fats and partially hydrogenated fats such as margarine and shortening are the worst forms of fat for the brain. These fats are found in most cookies, pastries, cakes, pies and other baked goods. These fats have been transformed into a trans fatty acid, which is a very destructive form of fat. These dangerous fats can interfere with normal cellular function in the brain.

Most Americans use margarine, which is the most destructive form of fat that we can consume. Many peanut butters purchased in grocery stores contain high amounts of hydrogenated fats.

If your child's diet includes peanut butter sandwiches, pastries, cakes, pies, cookies and margarine, these dangerous fats could be affecting their brain cells. These foods can negatively impact your child's ability to learn, focus and maintain attention.

The Good Guys

Monounsaturated fats are healthy fats for cell membranes. These good guys also protect against free-radical reactions. Here's a list of monounsaturated you should use often:

- Olive oil
- Macadamia nut oil
- Canola oil

Monounsaturated fats are also found in olives, avocados, almonds and macadamia nuts.

Omega-3 fats. The healthiest fats for the brain are the Omega-3 fatty acids. Omega-3 fatty acids are found in flaxseed oil and fish oils.

Understand that your brain is your body's fattiest organ. In fact, 60 percent of the brain is made up of lipids, which are fatlike substances. This is the reason that bad fats have such a negative impact on your child's ability to think and process information. Good fats have the opposite effect. The best fats for the brain are those found in fish oils.

Fish oils help prevent free-radical damage to

the brain cells. It also helps the cell membranes to become more pliable, which results in better communication between the synapses of the brain cells. This helps your brain function better.

Fish Is Brain Food

Brain cells and the myelin sheath, which is the protective covering around nerves, depend on assorted fats such as fish oil to function at peak efficiency. Intelligence is determined more by the number and quality of synapses rather than the number of brain cells. Fish oil is a primary building material for these synapses. The synapses enable nerve cells to communicate with one another and transmit these messages to other neurons.

You see, fish oil keeps the cell membranes of the brain cells soft and flexible so that neurotransmitter messages can get through.

Saturated fats create rigid cell membranes that hinder neurotransmitter communications. Let me explain how this works. Information travels from storage sites along a kind of electrical highway. Neurotransmitters are brain chemicals that have unique shapes. As these chemicals travel, receptor sites must receive them in the same way that a key unlocks a lock. When the membranes of your brain cells have a lot of Omega-3 fish oils (Omega-3 fatty acids), the membranes become soft and flexible. This allows the receptors to easily conform to the neurotransmitter's shapes. In other words, thoughts flow easily and freely through the brain.

But when receptors become rigid by eating the wrong kinds of fats, it becomes difficult for neurotransmitters to fit into receptor sites. Communication between cells is hindered or stopped altogether.

So you see, your child's brain may have plenty of neurotransmitters, but if the receptor sites are stiff and inflexible, thought messages will not flow easily through the brain.

Fish is "brain food," and the more fatty fish you can feed your child on a weekly basis the better off his brain will be. Serve fish to your family often. Cook salmon, mackerel, herring, tuna, sardines or other fatty fish approximately two to three times a week.

Fried foods are also damaging to brain cells. When you prepare fish, grill, bake or broil it. If your child refuses to eat fish, try offering liquid flaxseed oil. It may be used as a salad dressing, added to a nutritional drink or taken as a supplement—1 tablespoon one to two times a day or one to two capsules three times a day with meals. We will discuss supplements your child can take in the next chapter.

Here's a great shake recipe that will help your child get the Omega-3 oil he needs.

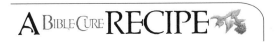

A BIBLE CURE RECIPE

TRY A BRAIN SHAKE

Start your child's day with a "brain shake." These brain-nourishing nutrients can help your child perform better in school.

    1 cup soy milk
    1 Tbsp. granular lecithin
    1 Tbsp. flaxseed oil
    1 heaping Tbsp. soy protein powder, such
        as Prozone Vegetarian Protein Powder (This is
        a forty-thirty-thirty protein powder, which can
        be found at many health food stores.)

Blend these ingredients together. Add crushed ice or any frozen fruit that has not been packed in syrup.

Give your child this shake after breakfast and when he returns home from school.

Food Sensitivities and ADD

Many children with ADD and ADHD have multiple food sensitivities. These kids' behavior can dramatically improve when certain foods are identified and eliminated from their diets.

Some of the more common foods that hyperactive children are sensitive to include the following:

- Sugars
- Corn syrup
- Eggs
- Milk products
- Grains, especially wheat
- Junk food
- Food dyes
- Food preservatives
- Food additives
- Artificial colors
- Artificial sweeteners

A comprehensive food sensitivity test will often identify your child's food sensitivities. This test is not very expensive, and many insurance companies will pay for it. The Great Smokies Diagnostic Lab in Asheville, NC, performs this test. To find a doctor in your area, visit their website at www.gsdl.com. I also often recommend that

parents place their children on foods that are rec-
ommended for their blood type.

A new method of food allergy elimination is
called NAET. This is a painless method that
involves acupressure points. Many nutritional
doctors practice it. To find a doctor in your area,
visit their website at www.naet.com.

Additives, Preservatives and Caffeine

Some experts blame ADD and ADHD solely on food
additives, preservatives and salicylates.[1] Some
believe that eliminating artificial colorings, preservatives such as BHA and BHT and foods with natural salicylates (such as raisins, almonds, toma-
toes, oranges, apples, peaches and berries) will
improve your child's hyperactivity.[2]

Some children improve significantly from this
diet, but others do not. Eliminate these items
from your child's diet, as well as caffeinated products, and carefully watch to see if his symptoms
improve.

Intelligent Eating Plan

It is critically important to provide your child with
low-glycemic foods during the day at regular
intervals, approximately every three to four

hours, in order to keep the blood sugar stabilized. Avoiding high-glycemic foods, fruit juices, high-sugar desserts, candies, cookies, cakes and pies also helps.

Here's an example of a healthy breakfast, lunch and dinner for a child with ADD or ADHD.

Breakfast

By increasing protein during the day, such as meat, poultry, seafood, peas, beans, lentils and tofu, you can help to jump-start your ADD child's brain.

- Whole-grain, high-fiber cereal such as old-fashioned oatmeal or oat bran
- Piece of fruit
- Brain Shake

I also recommend a good vitamin and mineral supplement, which we will discuss in the next chapter.

Midmorning snack

Pack a midmorning snack in your child's backpack or lunch box. This will keep your child's blood sugar level from dropping too low or rising too high. This should consist of one of the following:

- Piece of fruit
- Balance Bar
- 40-30-30 nutritional snack

Lunch

A healthy lunch should consist of the following:

- Tuna or other fatty fish sandwich on whole-grain bread
- Lettuce
- Tomato
- Canola oil mayonnaise (which can be found at a health food store)
- Piece of fruit
- Skim or low-fat milk

Seafood, meat, poultry, lentils, peas, beans and tofu are also excellent foods to eat for lunch since they tend to stimulate the brain and help your child to focus.

After-school snack

It's important to have a balanced after-school snack ready for your ADD child when he returns home. After a snack, your ADD child will be able to do his homework with fewer distractions.

- Brain Shake
- Balance Bar
- Fruit

Dinner

You may increase the amount of carbohydrates at dinner. Offer desserts after dinner, but not after lunch or in the afternoon. Carbohydrates at dinner will help to increase your child's serotonin level, which will help him sleep better. Also, give your child whole fruits instead of juices, and include vegetables and whole grains.

Drinks

Drinking adequate water is excellent for your child. Divide your child's body weight in pounds by two, and have him drink that amount of water in ounces a day. If your child weighs 100 pounds, he should drink 50 ounces of water a day. If he dislikes water, add freshly squeezed lemons with a few drops of the herbal sweetener Stevia or Splenda.

Small amounts of skim milk may also be beneficial, just as long as he's not sensitive or allergic to milk.

Conclusion

Taking the time and effort to help your ADD child learn to enjoy a different way of thinking about food may seem difficult at first. But let's face it. It certainly beats the alternative of medicating your child with heavy drugs that may produce damaging side effects.

Decide to make a commitment to healthy eating for your child's sake. It won't be long before you will discover hundreds of ways to include your entire family in a new lifestyle of brain-healthy habits that will benefit all of you.

As you learn and develop new habits, ask God to help you. Never forget how much He loves your child and how much He loves you, too! He will give you the patience, discipline and wisdom you need. All you need to do is ask.

The Bible says, "And so I tell you, keep on asking, and you will be given what you ask for. Keep on looking, and you will find. Keep on knocking, and the door will be opened. For everyone who asks, receives. Everyone who seeks, finds. And the door is opened to everyone who knocks" (Luke 11:9–10).

> *Her children stand and bless her.*
> —Proverbs 31:28

Why not begin developing a new lifestyle of healthy eating habits today?

A BIBLE CURE PRAYER
FOR YOU

Dear Lord, I commit my child's ADD or ADHD to You. You made my child, and You know him well. Give me Your wisdom to provide the diet my child needs to succeed. Give me the wisdom to make these dietary changes in fun and interesting ways. Help my ADD child to have Your grace to accept these dietary changes. I thank You for my child. I know You gave him to me as a holy trust, and I commit to being the best parent I know how to be with Your divine help. Amen.

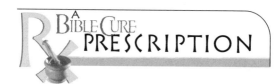

A BIBLE CURE PRESCRIPTION

Create an ADD/ADHD menu plan for your child.

Breakfast

_____

_____

_____

_____

Lunch

_____

_____

_____

_____

Dinner

_____

_____

_____

_____

Chapter 5

Success Through Supplements

Your child's brain and body are a masterful balance of artistry and chemistry, a perfect design of creative genius. God alone could create him. Your youngster was intricately and wonderfully made by Him! The Bible states:

> You made all the delicate, inner parts of my body and knit me together in my mother's womb. Thank you for making me so wonderfully complex! Your workmanship is marvelous—and how well I know it. You watched me as I was being formed in utter seclusion, as I was woven together in the dark of the womb.
> —PSALM 139:13–15

In His creative genius the divine Creator also supplied countless sources of energy to keep this wonderful creation working correctly. Vitamins and minerals are uniquely programmed by God to keep your child's mind and body functioning properly.

Today's fast-food lifestyles make it tough for your child to get all the nutrients he needs. In addition, you can provide powerfully beneficial supplements that will directly impact your child's ability to focus and process information. Let's take a look at a powerful brain-boosting program of vitamins, minerals, nutrients and other supplements that can change your youngster's life forever.

Vital Vitamins and Minerals

Multivitamin/multimineral. Start your child on a good comprehensive multivitamin and mineral formula that supplies the required daily allowances of vitamins and minerals. It should be taken daily.

Children eight years and older can usually swallow a whole-food multivitamin and mineral in capsule form. If a child cannot swallow a capsule, a chewable or liquid multivitamin may be used. It is, however, very difficult to get adequate vitamins and minerals in chewable or liquid multivitamins. Therefore I recommend that parents open the contents of a whole-food vitamin capsule and sprinkle it in applesauce and give it to their child two to three times a day. Divine Health whole-food vitamins are excellent.

Zinc. Children often have zinc deficiencies because the main sources for zinc include foods that many children don't like—foods such as eggs, seafood, nuts, seeds and whole-grain bread. Zinc deficiencies affect both learning and behavior. Check to be sure that your multivitamin contains zinc.

B-complex vitamins. Your child's behavior and ability to learn can also be affected when B-complex vitamins are lacking in his diet. A good multivitamin will also contain B-complex vitamins.

Iron. Most American children aren't getting enough iron in their diets. Without enough iron, your child's attention span can be decreased. Adolescent girls are especially vulnerable to deficiencies in iron.

A simple blood test can determine if your child needs iron. Ask your family physician or pediatrician to test your child for iron deficiency, especially if your youngster has been diagnosed with ADD and ADHD.

Lecithin. The brain-boosting nutrient choline has been proven to be extremely safe for children with ADD. Acetylcholine is an incredible neuro-transmitter and is the main brain chemical for thought and memory. You can purchase choline or phosphatidyl choline from any health food store. The best way to get enough choline is to take lecithin supplements.

Lecithin supplements are very inexpensive, easy to digest and completely nontoxic. They are available in liquid, capsule, granules, powder and tablet form. I recommend the capsule and granular forms mainly.

Take 2000 to 3000 milligrams three to four times a day. Children under twelve years of age need only half this amount, or about 1000 to 1500 milligrams, three to four times a day.

> *Those who fear the LORD are secure; he will be a place of refuge for their children.*
> —PROVERBS 14:26

Another way to get lecithin is to drink a chlorophyll drink such as Green Super Food from Divine Health Nutritional Products, which contains high amounts of lecithin.

Vitamin C. In order for your body to transform lecithin into the neurotransmitter acetylcholine, it requires plenty of vitamins C and B_5, which is pantothenic acid.

Vitamin C, B_5, lecithin and a good multivitamin will help assure that your child has plenty of acetylcholine, which will help him to focus, improve his memory and learn more efficiently.

Take 500 milligrams of vitamin C three times a day for children over twelve. Take 250 milligrams three times a day for children under twelve. If your child experiences an upset stomach, diarrhea or any other side effects, simply lower the dosage.

Vitamin B_5. Children over twelve usually need at least 100 milligrams of B_5 per day, and children under twelve need approximately 50 milligrams of B_5 per day. B_5 is very safe. Again, it is best to take this two to three times a day instead of taking it all at once.

B-complex, which includes all eight B vitamins, vitamin C and magnesium can all be taken in a comprehensive multivitamin and mineral capsule or tablet.

Don't place your children on amino acids, even though they can be purchased at a health food store. Phenylalanine and tyrosine are amino acids that are converted to the neurotransmitter norepinephrine, which may help to focus. It is important to be under the care of a nutritional doctor to monitor these supplements.

Fish oil. I recommend DHA/EPA supplements (fish oil) in gel capsule form with added vitamin E to prevent rancidity. Fish oil capsules should contain about 120 milligrams of DHA and 180 milligrams of EPA. Take one capsule three times a day with meals.

Flaxseed oil. I also recommend flaxseed oil taken in capsule or liquid form, approximately 1 tablespoon, one to two times a day. Or take one to two of these gel capsules three times a day with meals.

Building
Brainpower With DMAE

Another nutrient called DMAE (otherwise known as dimethylaminoethanol) helps raise production of acetylcholine, especially when it is taken with B_5.

DMAE is found in some seafood, especially sardines. This is one of the reasons why seafood is called brain food.

DMAE can help improve learning and memory. It is also able to help with learning problems that are associated with ADD. Start your child on low dosages of DMAE only under the supervision of a nutritional doctor.

Start with 50 milligrams twice a day. Children under twelve should start with 25 milligrams twice a day. If your child feels overstimulated, you may need to decrease the dosage.

One hundred milligrams twice a day is an effective dose. Build up to this level gradually. Generally it will take a few weeks to notice an improvement in your child's focus, memory and behavior.

By providing a regular regimen of vitamins, minerals and supplements, you will give your ADD child's brain what it needs to function in a healthier, more focused way.

Conclusion

God doesn't want you to go through one more painful day of watching your child struggle to complete homework, interact with others and struggle to succeed. Never forget that God created your youngster, and He knows exactly what your child needs. God's love for your child is much greater than your own. He will help you to help your ADD child.

A BIBLE CURE PRAYER
FOR YOU

Lord, I'm thankful that You created my child with Your own creative genius. You made him truly unique and special, according to Your own awesome plan. I choose to trust You to be with my ADD youngster throughout his journey and to bring him to the joyful purpose of Your plan for him. Your plan for my ADD child is truly awesome, and it started when You formed him in the womb. Equip his mind and body to function at optimal level. Teach him discipline and patience. Thank You, God, that my child will succeed in all that You put before him because of Your loving grace upon him. Amen.

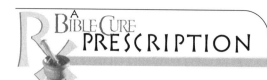

A BIBLE CURE PRESCRIPTION

Write out your own uniquely tailored vitamin, mineral and supplement plan based upon the information in this chapter.

_____

_____

_____

_____

_____

_____

Write a prayer thanking God for your child, for his destiny and for His help in getting him there.

_____

_____

_____

_____

_____

_____

Chapter 6

Faith
for Fulfillment

Faith is the power of God in action through His wonderful and mighty Word. But did you know that love is the key that unlocks faith's door? The Bible says, "The important thing is faith—the kind of faith that works through love" (Gal. 5:6, NCV).

The power of faith is released in your child's life when it is touched by love. The love you have for your child is a force that will get him through his struggles with ADD or ADHD. The love that God has for both of you will be an invisible hand strengthening, supporting and comforting you.

God has not forgotten about your child. He knows his every need, his every thought, his every fear and problem. Neither has God forgotten you! The Bible says that you and your child are the apple of God's eye. (See Zechariah 2:8). His favor, affection and love are poured out from heaven toward you, even at this very moment.

God promises to get you through this difficulty:

> When you go through deep waters and great trouble, I will be with you. When you go through rivers of difficulty, you will not drown! When you walk through the fire of oppression, you will not be burned up; the flames will not consume you. For I am the LORD, your God, the Holy One of Israel, your Savior . . . you are precious to me. You are honored, and I love you.
>
> —ISAIAH 43:2–4

Building Up Your Child in Faith and Love

More important than nutrition or nutrient, supplement or lifestyle change, you can build up your ADD child in the power of faith and love. Believe in God's love and the power of your own love for success, because the Bible says, "Love never fails" (1 Cor. 13:8, NAS).

Many children with ADD and ADHD have a low self-esteem and feel as if they are failures. The more failing grades and failing tests that your child receives, the more these fears are reinforced in his heart.

Building a strong sense of self-esteem within your child will give him a lifelong shield of defense. Here are some helpful hints:

- Start with small success stories. Praise his accomplishments, no matter how small. Has he completed a homework assignment? Has he make a good grade on a test? Praise him heartily for his success.

- Sometimes it may be very difficult to find anything about which to praise your child. Nevertheless, it's critically important to find something positive to praise your child for.

- Praise your child every day and often.

Healing a Wounded Spirit

ADD kids are very vulnerable to being wounded. It's easy for them to begin seeing life through a feeling of rejection, failure and defeat. You can protect your child from deep wounds of the spirit. The Bible says, "The human spirit can endure a sick body, but who can bear it if the spirit is crushed?" (Prov. 18:14).

These children tend to be extremely sensitive, and defeat, no matter how small, just reinforces

71

their wounded sense of failure. But you can break them out of a negative belief system through daily encouragement and praise.

As you build up your ADD child with praise, eventually he will begin to believe he is a success. A little encouragement will fill his heart with new courage. He will study harder to receive more praise. So you can see how praise breaks a cycle of defeat and failure and begins to replace it with an upward spiral of success and joy.

Your ADD child needs praise throughout each and every day. Once his grades improve, you must not let up. If your encouragement wanes, he will tend to regress back to his old negative belief system that tells him he can't do it. Small success leads to greater successes and a good academic self-image. But if your child always feels that he is behind all the other children, it's easy for him to become discouraged and give up.

Your Attitude and Your ADD Child's Altitude

Your attitude toward your ADD child will determine how high up the ladder of personal success he will go. Encourage your ADD child through a caring, friendly and respectful attitude.

Try not to speak to him in a harsh, disapproving voice over inadequate grades and test scores. This will not encourage him to do better. It will discourage him and often may cause him to perform worse than before.

I want to emphasize again that these children are very sensitive. If they are not encouraged in a loving, compassionate way, they will likely reject your counsel and will become more discouraged.

Shielding Your
ADD Child From Labels

Many children with ADD get labeled: brat, stupid, lazy, stubborn, spacey, wild and crazy. Teachers and adults call these children ADD or hyperactive, which is an improvement in the label, but it still labels them as problem kids.

Consider choosing these attitude improvements:

- Instead of calling these kids hyperactive, why not simply say they are high-energy or spirited youngsters? This might help both teachers and parents to view them in a more positive way.

- Instead of seeing an ADD child as impulsive, see him as spontaneous.

- Instead of seeing your child as distract-ible, see him as creative.

- Instead of seeing him as a daydreamer, see him as imaginative.

- Instead of seeing your child as irritable, see him as sensitive.

Sometimes it's really tough to see another person in a new light, even if that individual is your own child. But by choosing your own more positive attitudes, you will create a more positive image of your child. His behavior will eventually begin to conform.

The Power of Your Words

Give your child hope, and remove all the negative labels by speaking positive words over your child's life. Proverbs 18:21 says, "Death and life are in the power of the tongue, and those who love it will eat its fruit" (NAS). Ephesians 4:29 tells us that we are to "let no corrupt word proceed out of your mouth" (NKJV).

Realize that if we speak out of our mouths that our children are brats, irritable, hyperactive, lazy or stupid, then we will reap the harvest of those words.

But if we speak those positive things that we truly believe are within our children, eventually their behavior will conform to our words. As parents we must walk in love according to John 13:34–35:

> A new commandment I give to you, that you love one another; as I have loved you, that you also love one another. By this all will know that you are My disciples, if you have love for one another.
>
> —NKJV

Passing Your Parent Test

ADD children may test your love and patience more than many other children. But you are up to the test, and God will help you to pass it. If you lean on Him daily and pray about each difficulty, you'll begin to see God's wonderful divine hand steadying your rocking boat, calming the stormy seas and bringing you to a joyful harbor. You will pass your ADD parent test!

Love never fails, and your love for your ADD child will make all the difference in the world.

God commands us to walk in love, and He will give our hard, empty hearts the power of love that we need to fulfill His command. Love is the strongest force in the universe, and when you walk in love, you walk in God.

The Greatest Force of All

First Corinthians 13 teaches us all about the characteristics of love. It says:

> Love is patient, love is kind and is not jealous; love does not brag and is not arrogant, does not act unbecomingly; it does not seek its own, is not provoked, does not take into account a wrong suffered, does not rejoice in unrighteousness, but rejoices with the truth; bears all things, believes all things, hopes all things, endures all things. Love never fails.
>
> —1 Corinthians 13:4–8, nas

If you are the parent of a child with ADD, this scripture must become *rhema*. That means it must become living, empowered truth in your life.

When both parents of an ADD child walk in the spirit of love, the spirit of strife, dissension and anger will eventually be removed from the home. The peace of God will dwell there. But when the law of love is broken, the home fills with strife, fighting, arguing and dissension, which makes the child's behavior worse.

The Power of a Merry Heart

Parents should practice a merry heart. According to Proverbs 17:22, "A merry heart does good, like medicine" (NKJV). Psalm 16:11 says, "In Your presence is fullness of joy" (NKJV). Nehemiah 8:10 says, "The joy of the LORD is your strength" (NKJV).

Create an atmosphere of laughter, love and peace in your home. You'll quickly discover that the spirit of strife and rebellion has been quenched.

Be Careful
Little Ears What You Hear

Children used to sing a little song in Sunday school that said, "Be careful little ears what you hear, for there's a God up above looking down on you with love." Most adults as well as children would do well to heed the words of this children's song.

If your child has ADD or ADHD, what he listens to is very important. Many children with ADD listen to rock-and-roll music or heavy metal, which is full of rebellion, defiance and anger. This kind of music can set an atmosphere in your home that's impossible to deal with.

It is critically important to play Christian music in the home, especially worship and praise music. Make your home a sanctuary of peace and love. This is only possible when both parents choose to walk in love.

Conclusion

ADD does not rule your home. The peace and love of God rule your home when you invite Him in. I encourage you to ask God for help in your family's struggle with ADD. He is as close as the whisper of a prayer. He will not fail you, nor will He ignore your request. He loves your family more than you can ever begin to imagine— every one of you, including you! If you open your heart to Him, you'll discover that He is a shelter in every storm, a strength in every battle and a loving Father. His ear is open to your prayer right now.

A BIBLE CURE PRAYER
FOR YOU

Dear Lord, I thank You that You love my family and that You love me. Thank You that in every situation, You have the answer. Your wisdom is greater than all my questions. With Your help each day, I commit to raising my ADD child in Your Bible cure way. I receive Your wisdom, patience and love to deal with each daily struggle. I receive a fresh vision of my child through Your eyes of hope, faith, love and success! Amen.

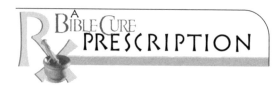

A BIBLE CURE PRESCRIPTION

What are the most challenging issues of faith and love that you are facing with your ADD child?

_____

_____

List five scriptures from this booklet that have inspired you to look to God for help.

_____

_____

Place these scriptures on your refrigerator, bathroom mirror or work area at your job to remind you to look to God. (circle one)

    I will   I probably won't do that

Write a prayer explaining to God your greatest challenges as a parent of an ADD child.

_____

_____

_____

A PERSONAL NOTE

From Don and Mary Colbert

God desires to heal you of disease. His Word is full of promises that confirm His love for you and His desire to give you His abundant life. His desire includes more than physical health for you; He wants to make you whole in your mind and spirit as well through a personal relationship with His Son, Jesus Christ.

If you haven't met my best friend, Jesus, I would like to take this opportunity to introduce Him to you. It is very simple.

If you are ready to let Him come into your heart and become your best friend, just bow your head and sincerely pray this prayer from your heart:

Lord Jesus, I want to know You as my Savior and Lord. I believe You are the Son of God and that You died for my sins. I also believe You were raised from the dead and now sit at the right hand of the Father praying for me. I ask You to forgive me for my sins and change my heart so that I can

be Your child and live with You eternally.
Thank You for Your peace. Help me to
walk with You so that I can begin to know
You as my best friend and my Lord. Amen.

If you have prayed this prayer, we rejoice with you in your decision and your new relationship with Jesus. Please contact us at pray4me@strang.com so that we can send you some materials that will help you become established in your relationship with the Lord. You have just made the most important decision of your life. We look forward to hearing from you.

Notes

CHAPTER 1
UNDERSTANDING ADD

1. *Diagnostic and Statistical Manual of Mental Disorders,* fourth edition (Washington, DC: American Psychiatric Association, 1994).

CHAPTER 2
LIFESTYLE SOLUTIONS

1. Source obtained from the Internet: Transcript from "A.D.D.—A Dubious Diagnosis," *The Merrow Report,* www.pbs.org/merrow/repository/Television/Past/_attn/add; "A Special Investigative Report on Ritalin," www.breggin.com/merrow.
2. Source obtained from the Internet: Parents Against Ritalin, www.p-a-r.org/concerns.

CHAPTER 3
EXERCISING OPTIONS

1. For more information on the history of neurofeedback, read *A Symphony in the Brain* by Jim Robbins (New York: Atlantic Monthly Press, 2000).

CHAPTER 4
A NATURAL NUTRITIONAL APPROACH

1. Benjamin Feingold, *Why Your Child Is Hyperactive* (New York: Random House, 1975).
2. Ibid.

Don Colbert, M.D., was born in Tupelo, Mississippi. He attended Oral Roberts School of Medicine in Tulsa, Oklahoma, where he received a bachelor of science degree in biology in addition to his degree in medicine. Dr. Colbert completed his internship and residency with Florida Hospital in Orlando, Florida. He is board certified in family practice and has received extensive training in nutritional medicine.

If you would like more
information about natural and
divine healing, or information about
Divine Health Nutritional Products®,
you may contact
Dr. Colbert at:

DR. DON COLBERT

1908 Boothe Circle
Longwood, FL 32750
Telephone: 407-331-7007
(For ordering products only)

Dr. Colbert's website is
www.drcolbert.com.

Disclaimer: Dr. Colbert and the staff of Divine Health Wellness Center are prohibited from addressing a patient's medical condition by phone, facsimile or e-mail. Please refer questions related to your medical condition to your own primary care physician.

Divine Health
ADD Formula

Do you or your child suffer the effects of attention deficit disorder and hyperactivity? God has a divine plan to help you overcome this condition. Divine Health ADD Formula is a healthy alternative to today's traditional method of treatment.

The herbs in this formula are intended to calm and relax. We recommend this blend of vitamins and herbs as a more natural alternative for the treatment of attention deficit disorder. We have encapsulated magnesium, German chamomile flowers, oat straw stem extract, valerian root and many other herbs in a small capsule for use with children as well as adults.

Product # 033 100 capsules $15.00

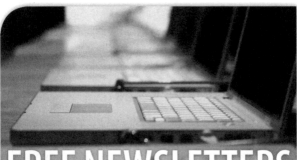